This book is dedicated to all those affected by Alzheimer's disease

Luke and his parents drove to the park to meet Grandpa Charles for ice cream.

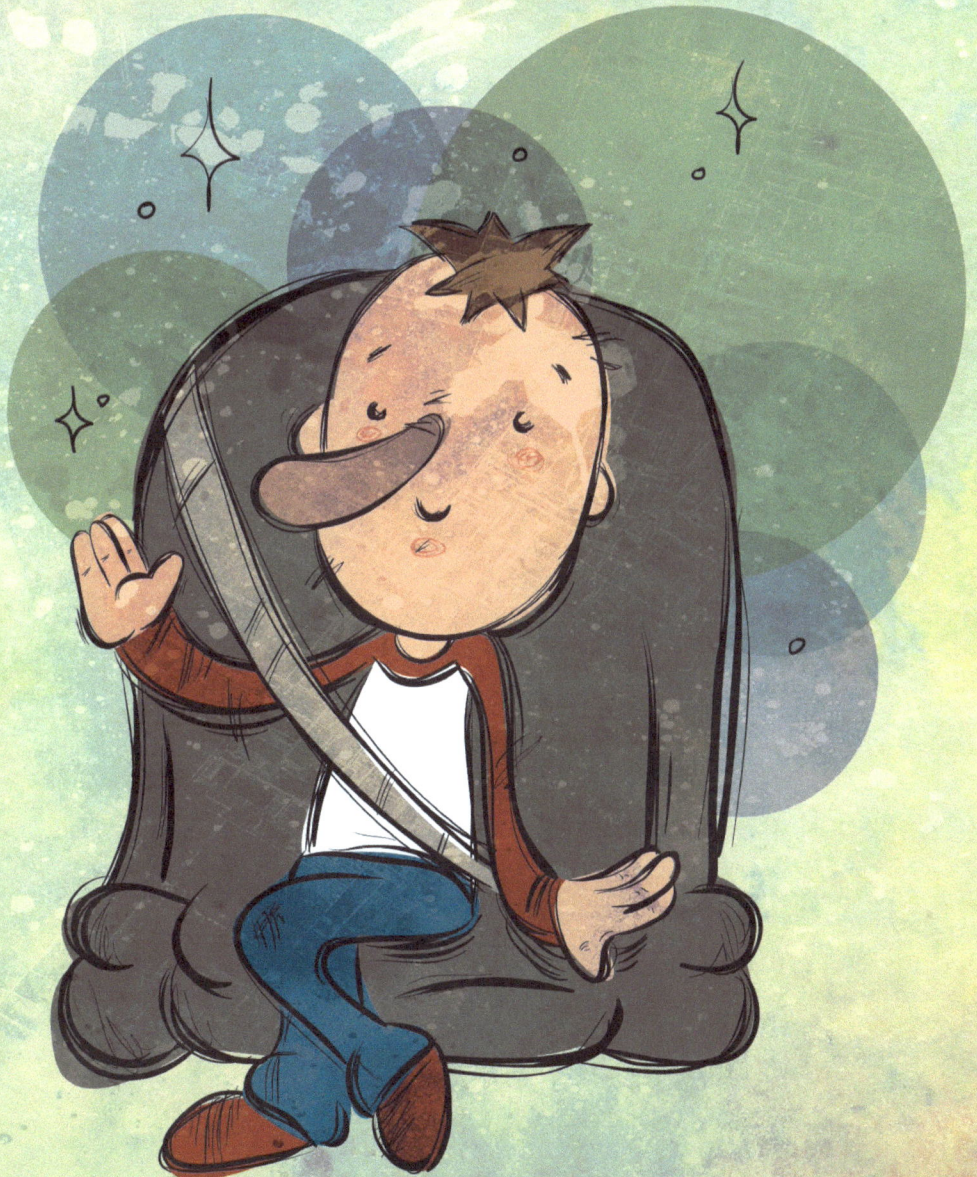

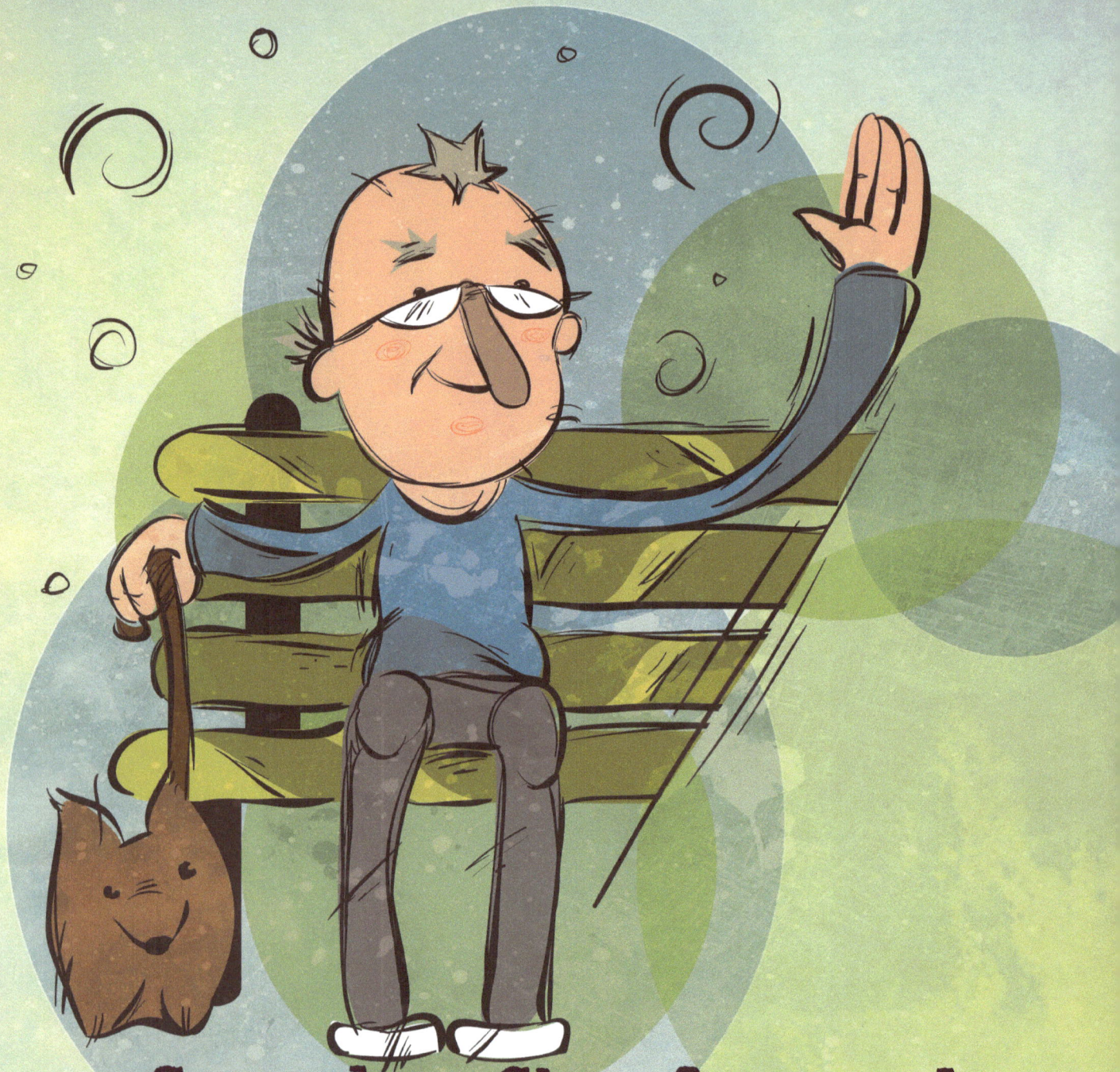

Grandpa Charles and his tiny dog Lilly sat on a bench near the ice cream cart.

Luke gave his grandpa a big hug and said, "Did you bring them? We have to toss them into the fountain! It's our tradition."

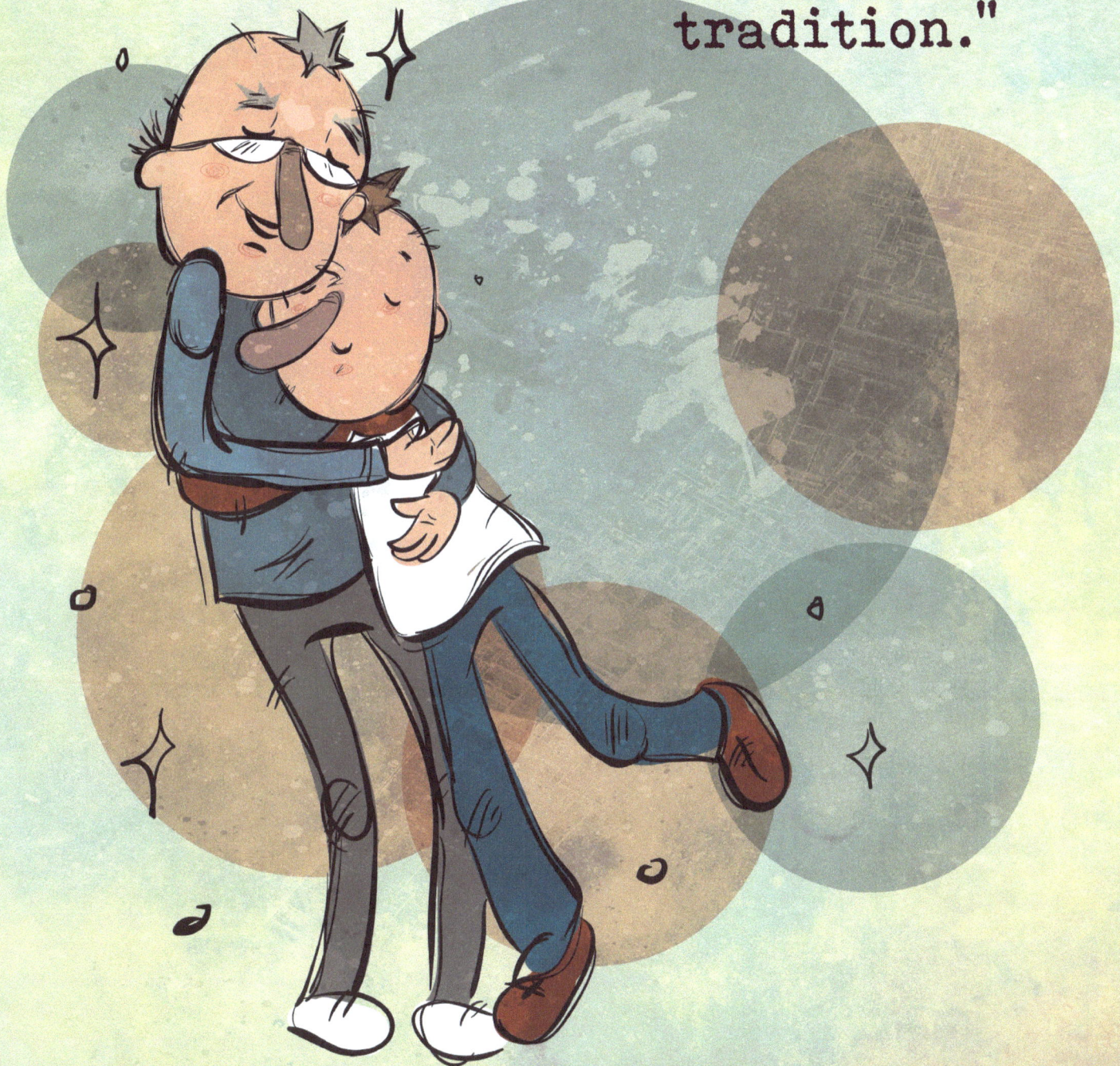

Grandpa Charles pulled
four shiny quarters
out of his pocket.

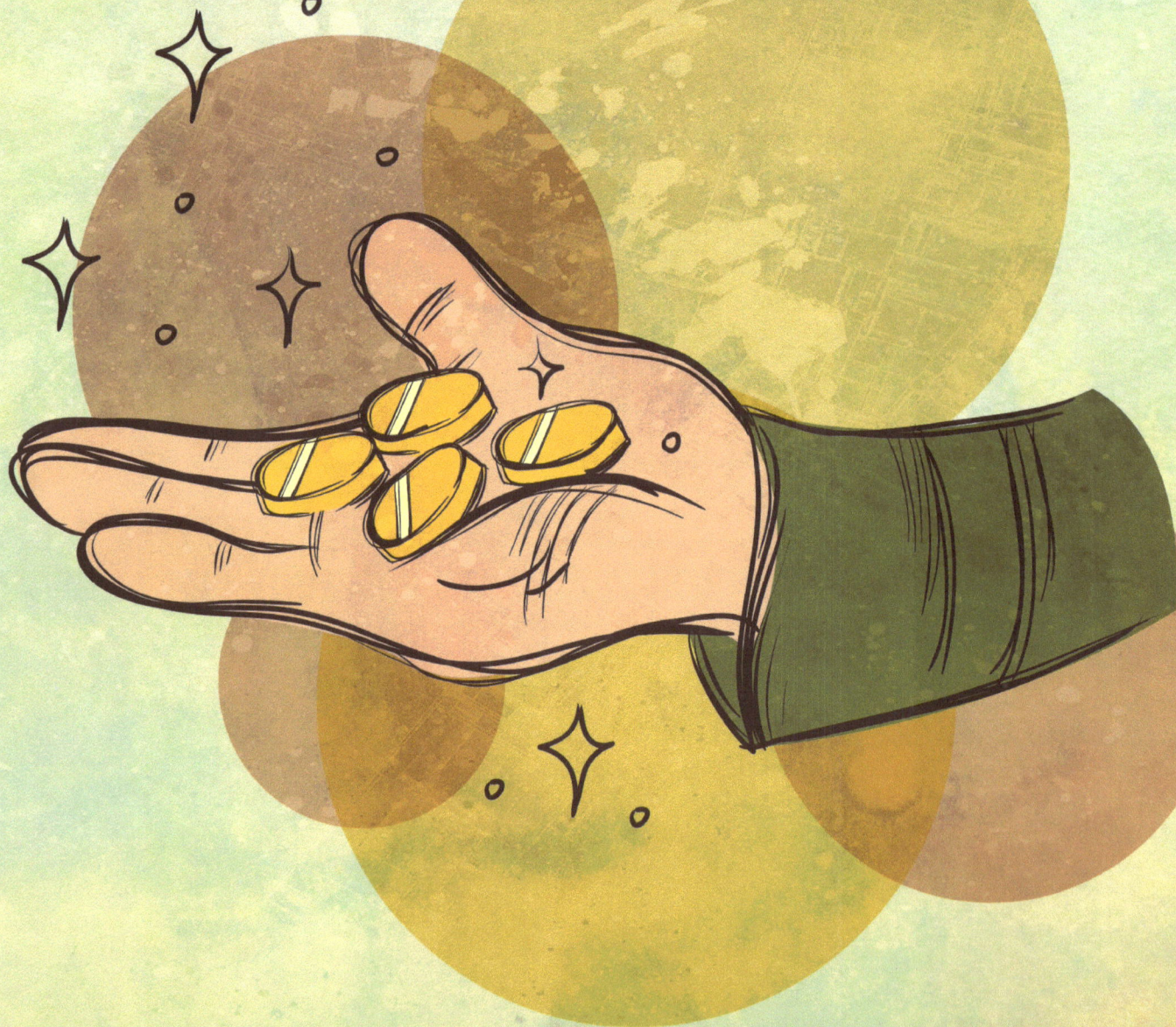

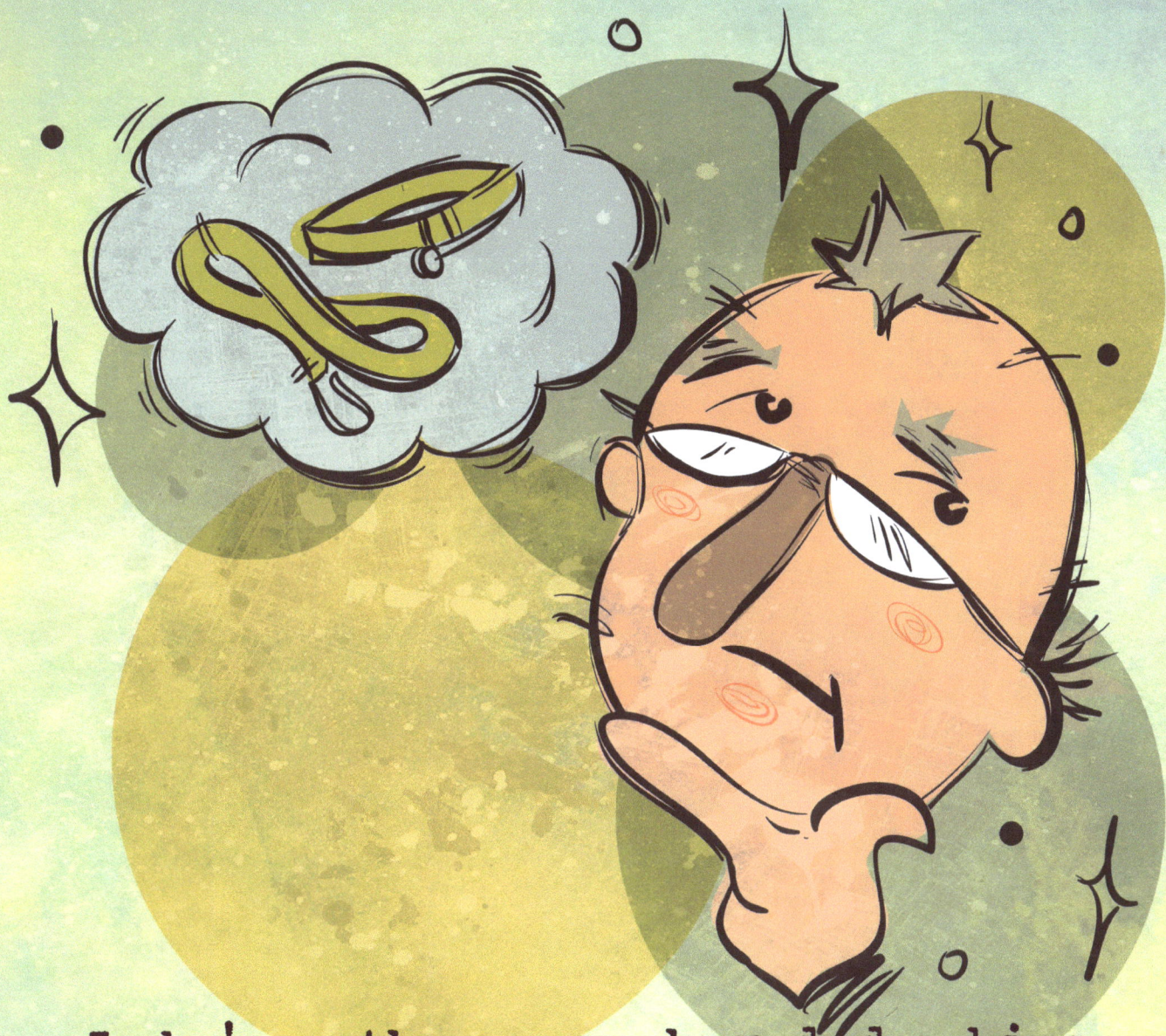

Luke's mother gave her dad a kiss
on the cheek then said, "Did you
have any difficulty getting to the
park, Dad?" He rubbed his chin and
said, "It took a while to find
Lilly's leash today."

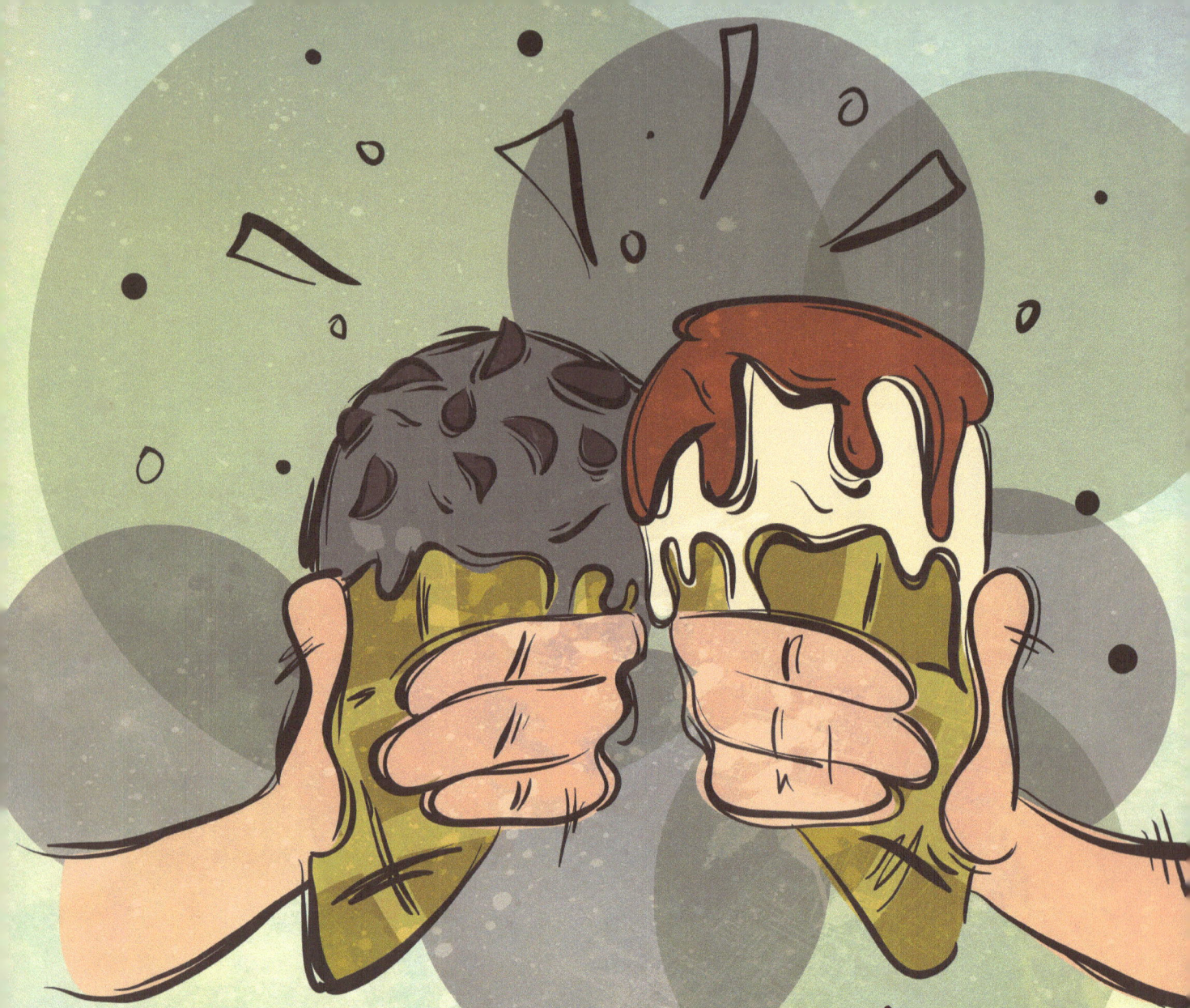

Luke tugged on his grandpa's sleeve and said, "Come on! Let's get some ice cream and make our way to the fountain. I have a special wish to make!"

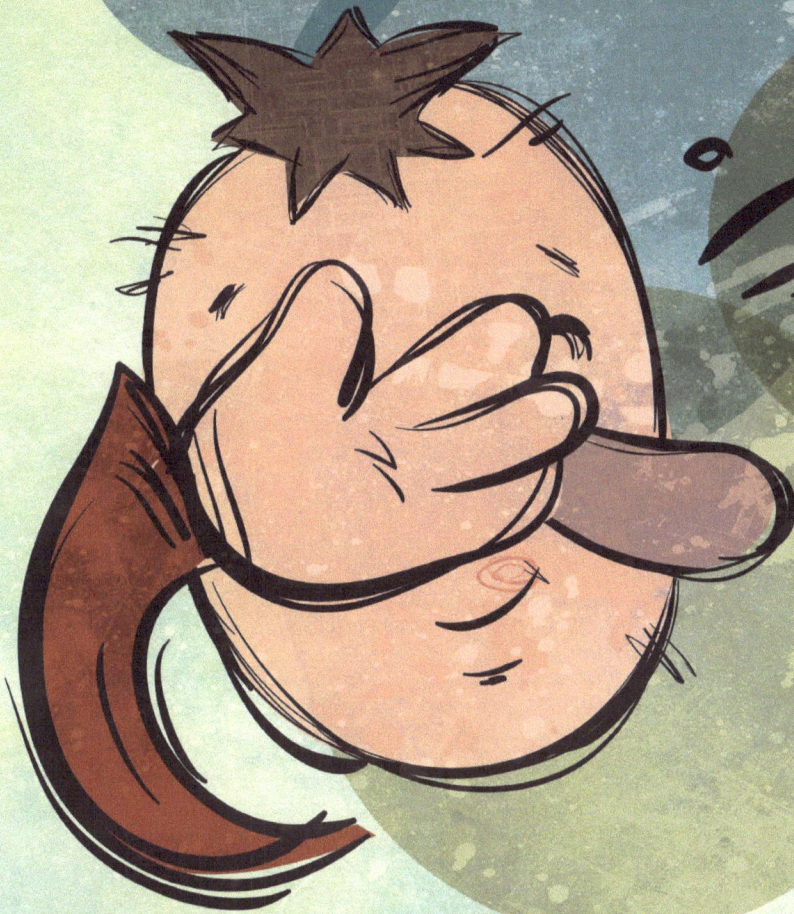

Grandpa Charles gave everyone a quarter. Luke closed his eyes tightly before flipping the quarter into the fountain. Grandpa Charles asked, "What did you wish for?" Luke responded, "I wished that I would score a goal in tomorrow's soccer game."

Luke asked his mom what she wished for. She responded, "I wished that everyone in this family stays good and healthy." She rubbed her dad's back as he cleaned his glasses with a tissue.

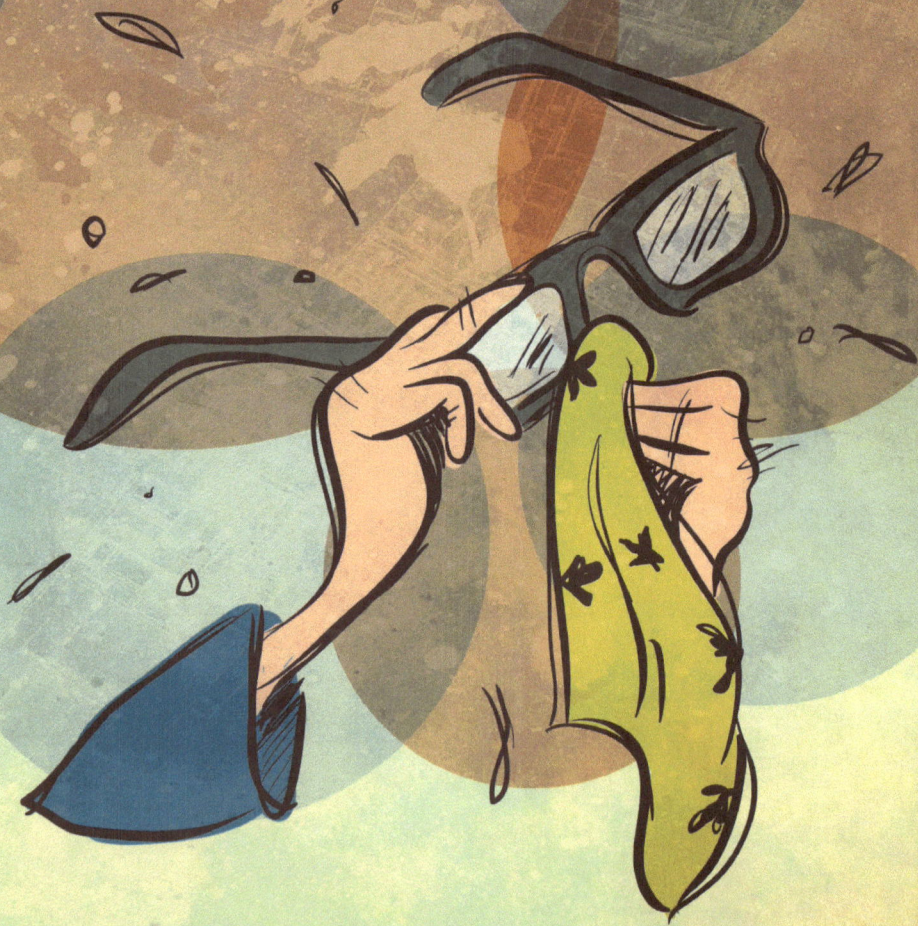

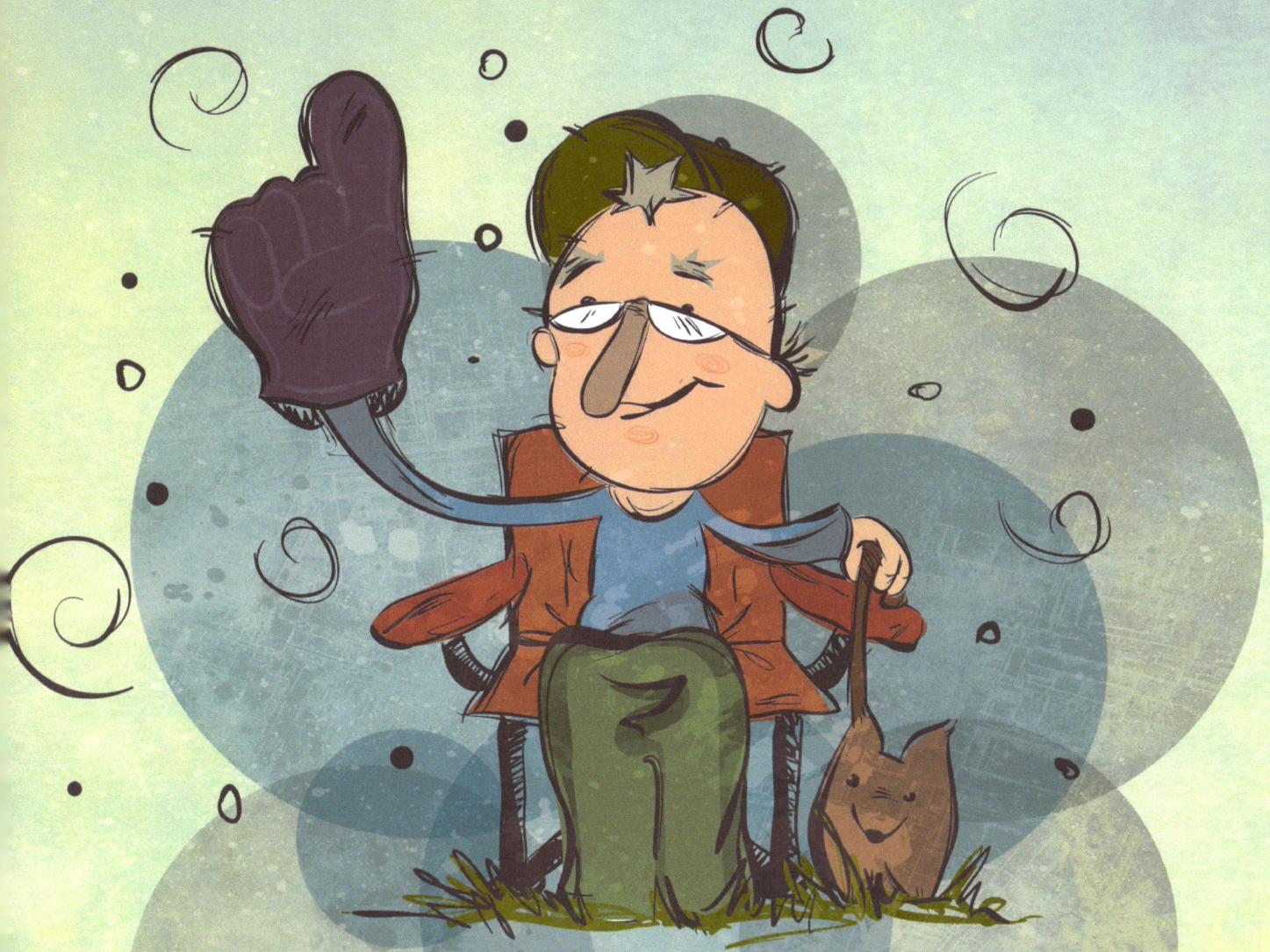

The next day Luke tightened the straps on his shin guards. Grandpa Charles loved watching Luke's soccer games. He was his grandson's biggest fan.

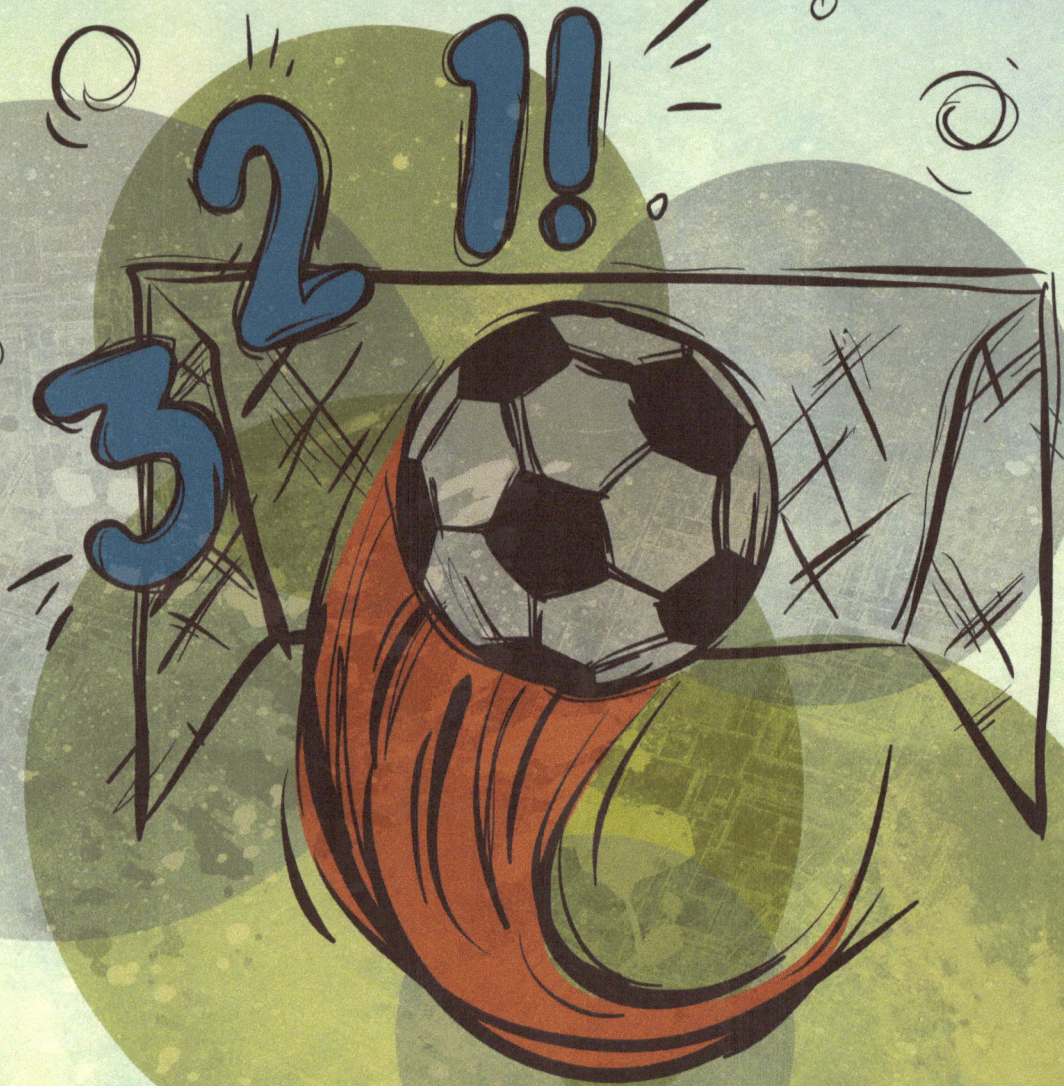

In the final seconds of the game Luke stole the soccer ball and raced down the field. Luke dribbled the ball between two defenders. The parents and fans of both teams counted down the clock, "3...2...1..." Luke kicked the ball as hard as he could and scored!

Luke sprinted to give his grandpa a high five, but when he looked under the umbrella his grandpa wasn't there. Luke and his parents looked in the restrooms but Grandpa Charles wasn't inside. Luke shouted, "Look! There's Grandpa; he's waiting in line for the ice cream cart." Luke's mom asked, "Dad, are you okay? You can't just take off like that." Grandpa Charles smiled and said, "I had to use the restroom, but I saw the ice cream and wanted to buy some." Luke's mom hugged her dad and they all walked back to the soccer field.

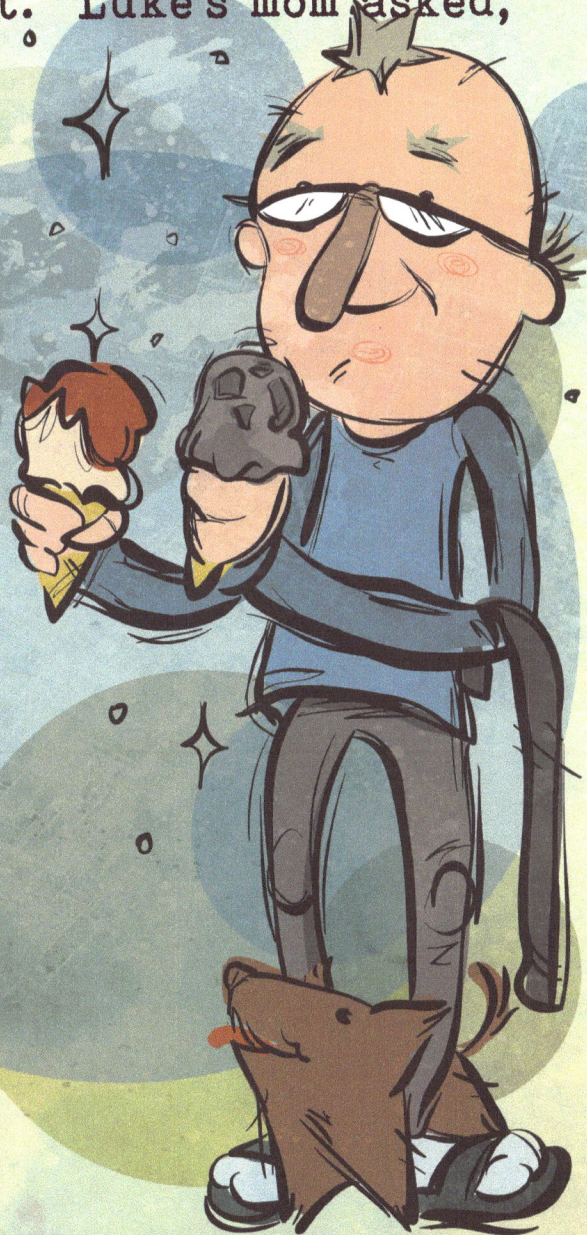

Grandpa Charles moved into an assisted living community in the fall. Luke was excited because now his grandpa lived even closer to his house. Luke asked his mom while they walked to visit Grandpa Charles, "So why did Grandpa move again?" She replied, "Your grandpa has Alzheimer's disease and he needs to live in a place where nurses and doctors can take care of him. He just can't live by himself anymore, but I'm sure he'll make new friends and of course he has us to visit."

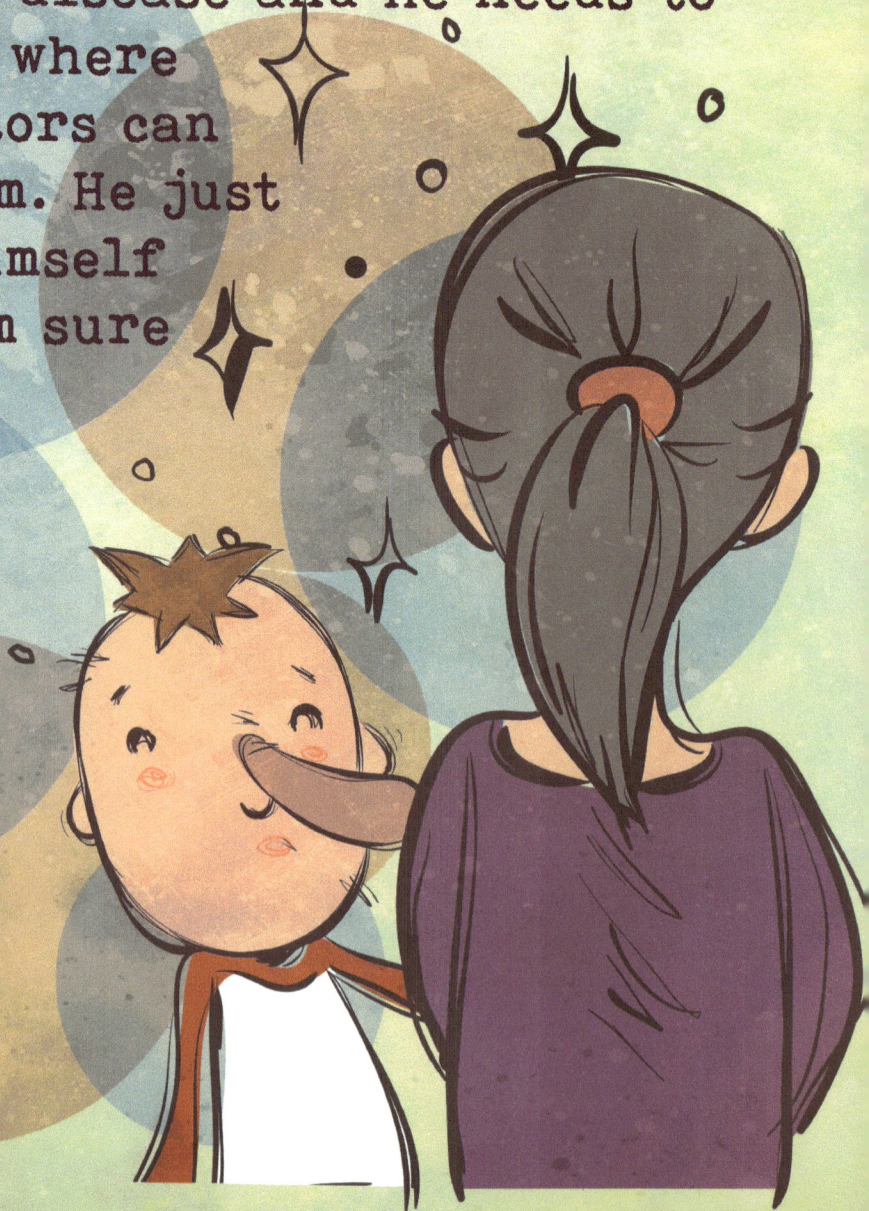

They entered a building called Memory Lane. Luke and his mom were greeted by a very nice nurse, "You must be here to see Grandpa Charles! He's a wonderful man. I think everyone's in the craft room making Halloween decorations."

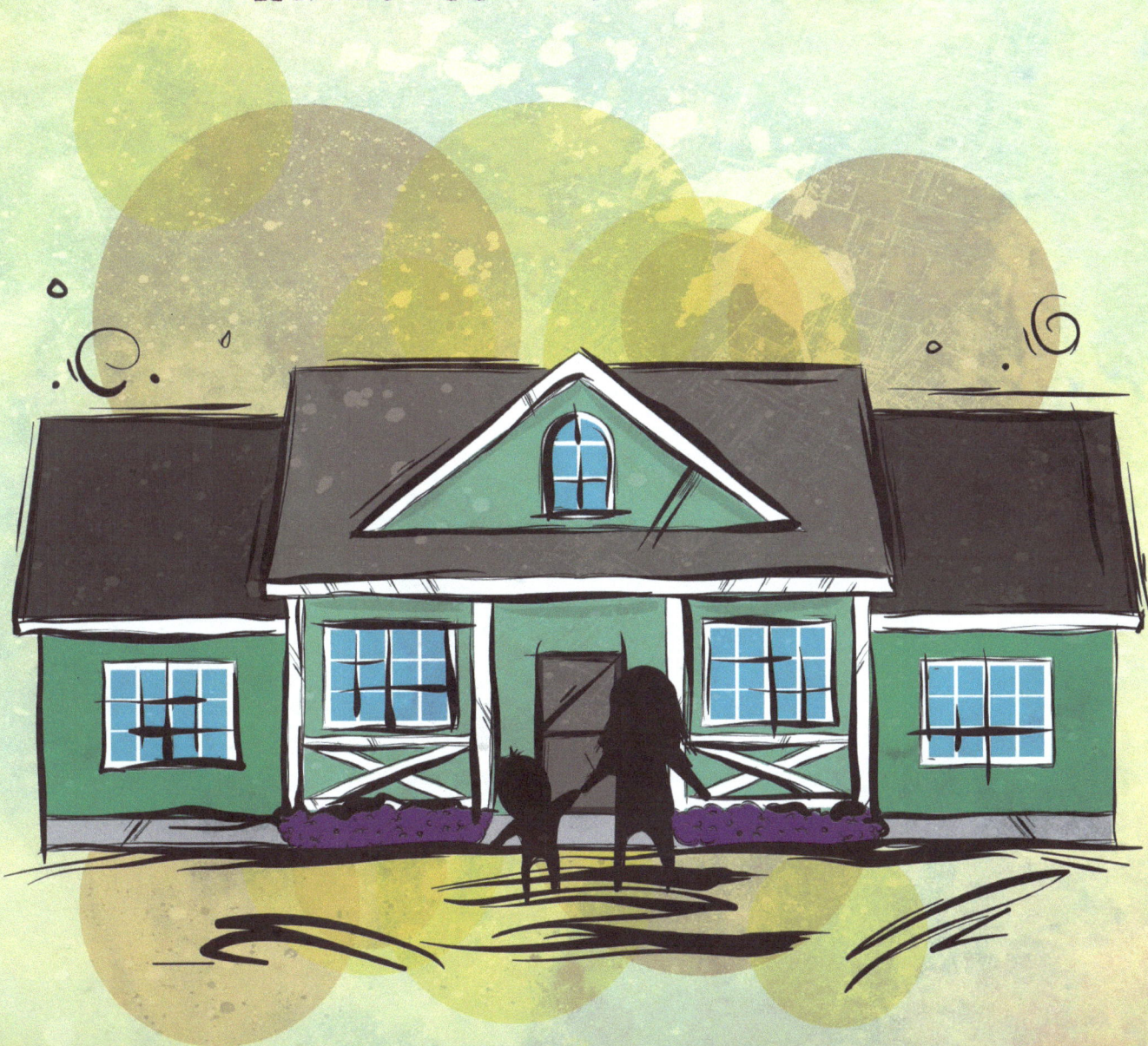

Luke ran to his grandpa's side and gave him a hug. He asked, "What are you painting, Grandpa?" Grandpa Charles took a moment and responded enthusiastically, "Yes!" Luke asked, "Is that a Frankenstein?" Grandpa Charles smiled and said, "Yes!"

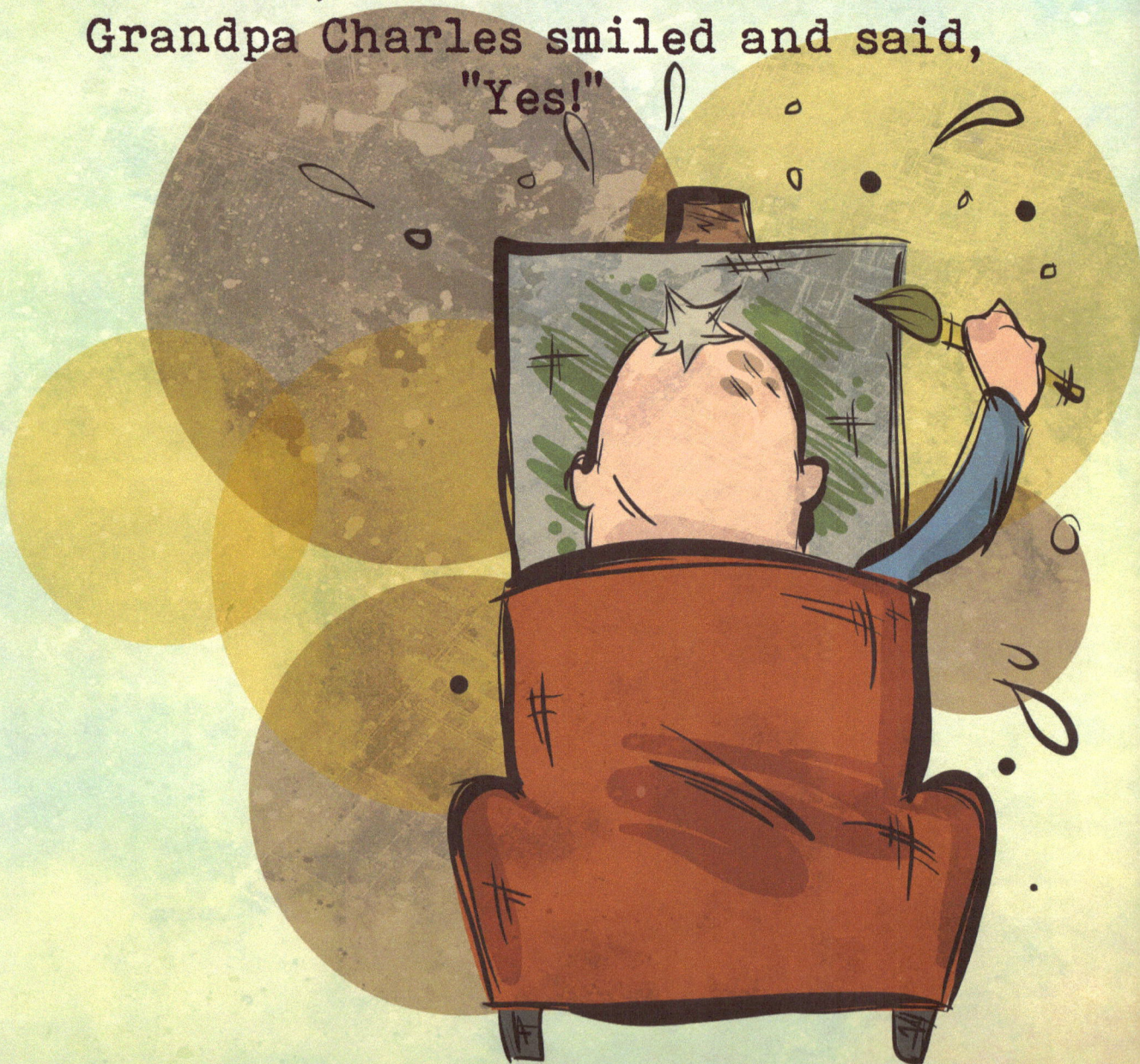

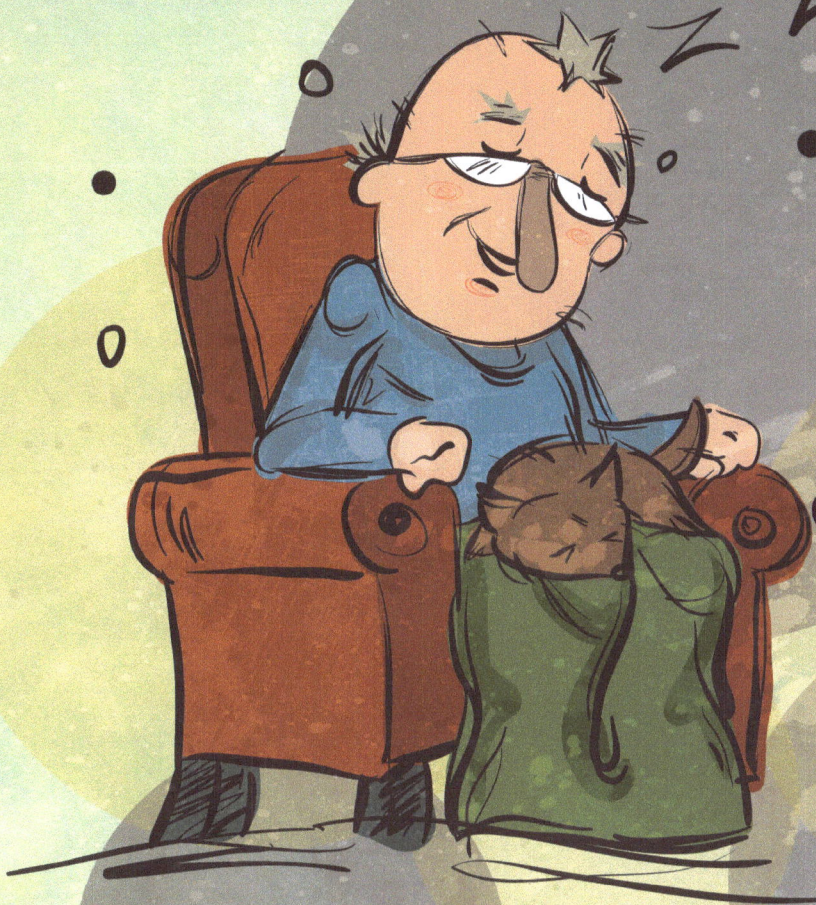

Luke and his mom played a card game while Grandpa Charles napped in a lounge chair with Lilly resting on his lap. Luke's mom said, "Aright, Luke, it's time to go." She pulled up the blanket, covering her father a little more and said, "Love you, Dad. We're going to take off, but we'll be back next weekend."

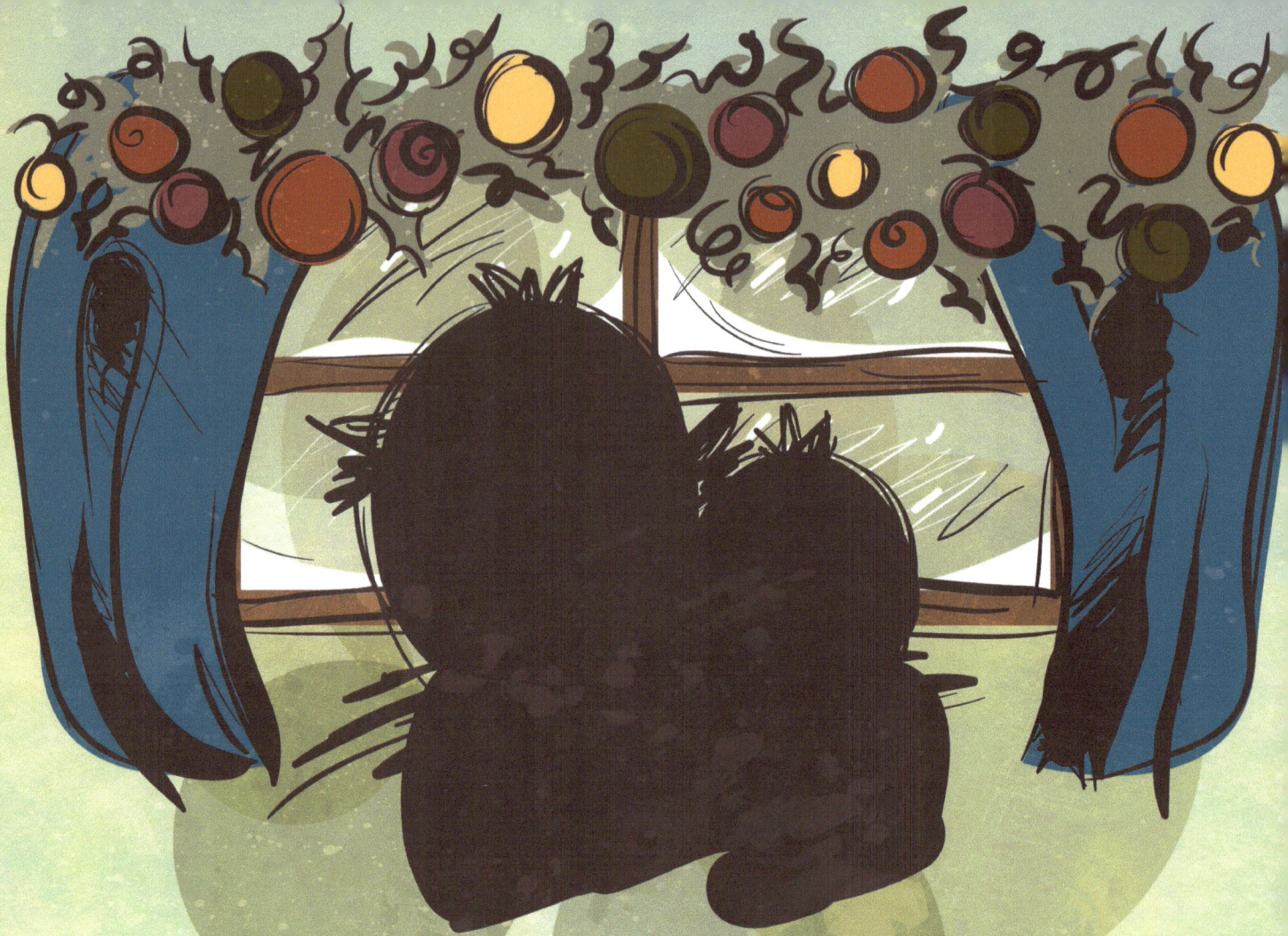

Snow piled up in the courtyard of
Memory Lane. "Look at all that
snow, Grandpa!" Luke said happily.
Grandpa Charles sat on a comfortable
couch near the window and said, "Yes!"
Luke sat next to him and they both
watched as a gentle snowfall
coated the furniture
outside.

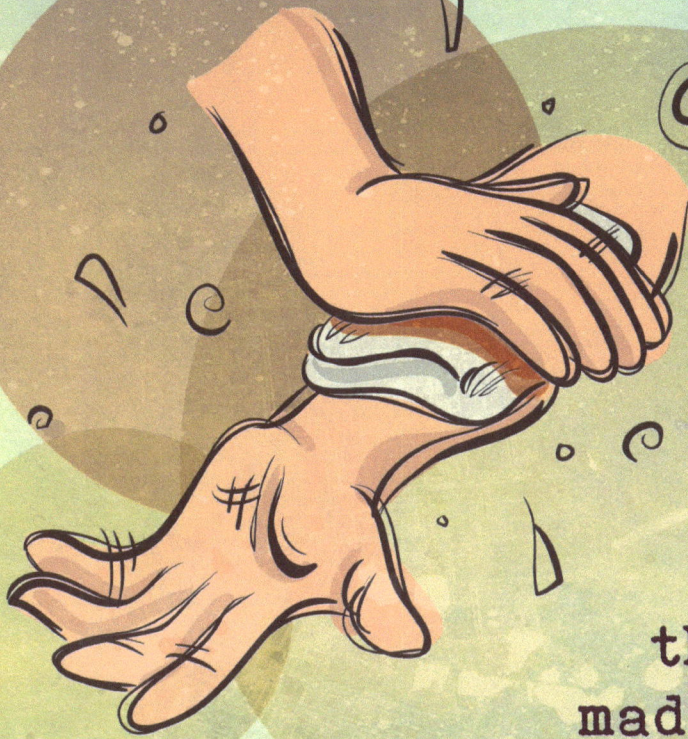

Luke couldn't wait to give Grandpa Charles his Christmas present. "Mom, do you think Grandpa will like the photo collage I made him?" She turned to Luke and said, "Oh yes! He's going to love it." They entered his bedroom where a nurse was dressing a bandage on Grandpa Charles's forearm. Luke's mother asked, "What happened?" The nurse responded, "Your father banged his arm on the dresser." Luke asked his grandpa, "Are you okay, Grandpa?" Grandpa Charles held out his hand and said, "Yes!"

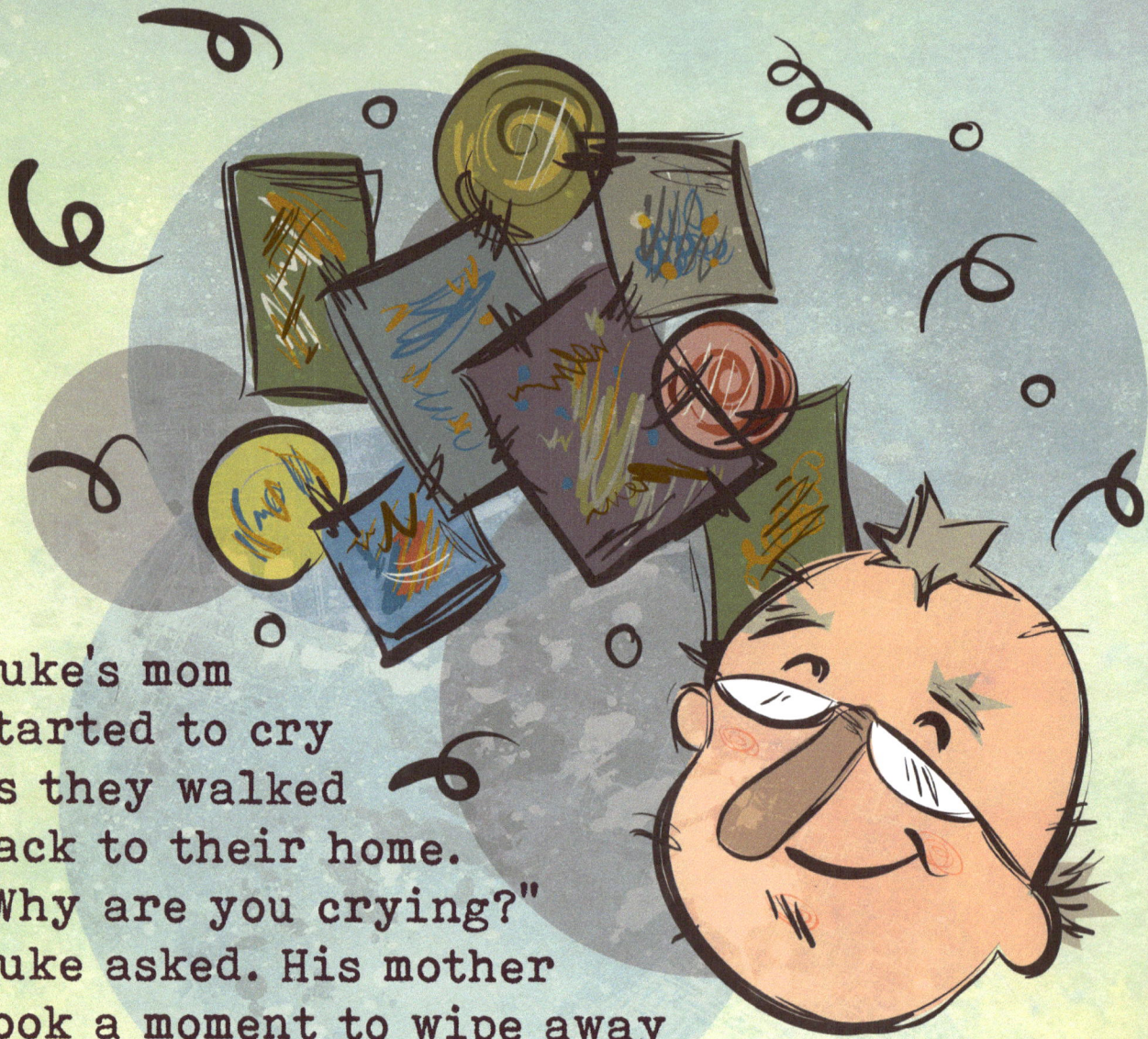

Luke's mom
started to cry
as they walked
back to their home.
"Why are you crying?"
Luke asked. His mother
took a moment to wipe away
her tears and said, "It's just
difficult seeing someone you love
in pain." Luke hugged his mom and
replied, "It's okay. Did you see how happy
Grandpa was to see us? He kept pointing
to the collage and smiling. This was a
good day and Grandpa Charles loved every
minute we visited."

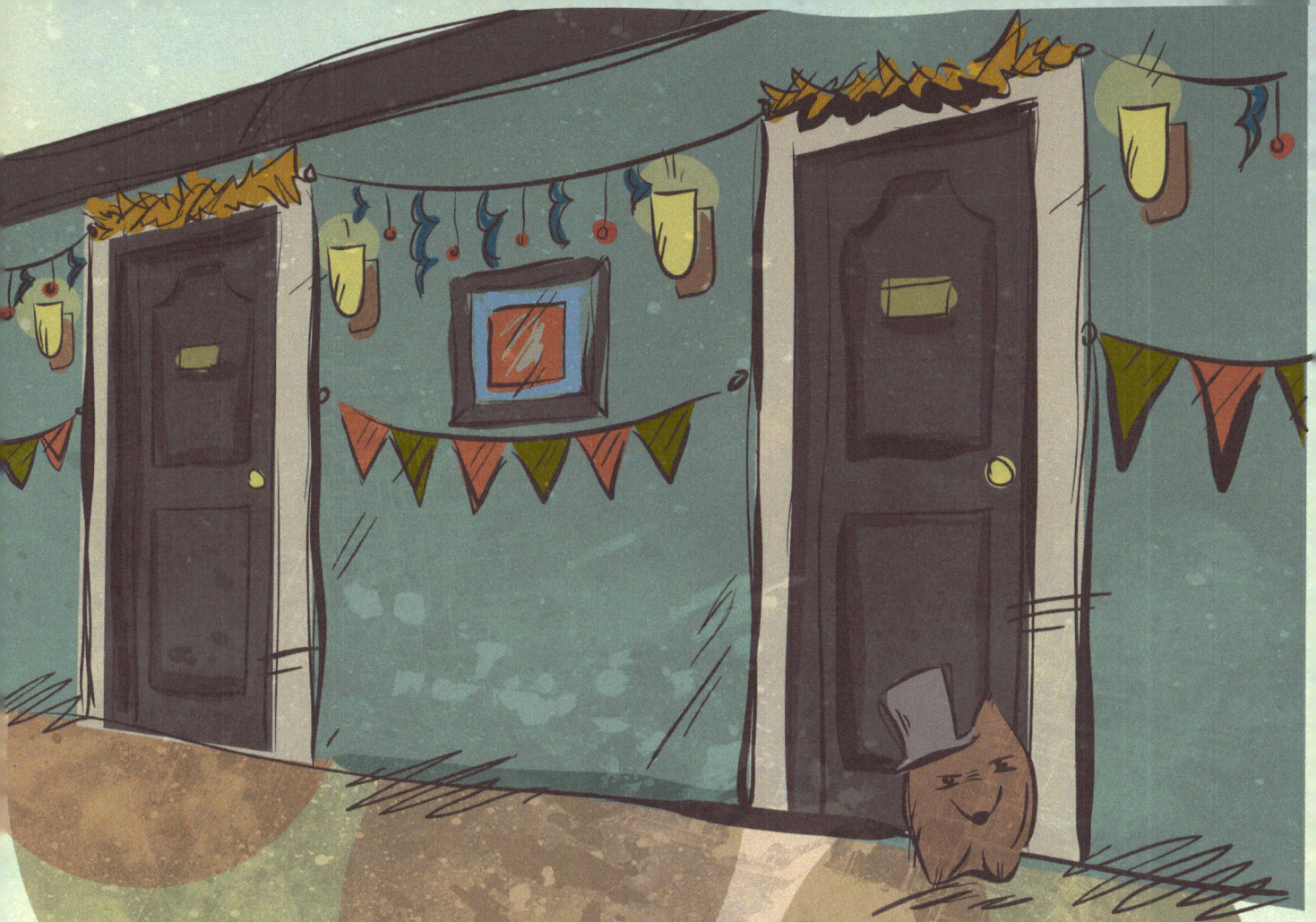

Memory Lane was decorated with
New Year's Eve posters. Luke placed
a small top hat on Lilly's head.
Grandpa Charles picked Lilly up
then sat in a chair to rest for a
moment.

Luke yawned then asked his mom a question while they watched the New Year's Eve celebrations on television, "Why is Grandpa so tired all the time?" She explained, "Your grandfather worked hard his entire life; this is his time to relax and rest. Speaking of rest, time for bed, kiddo."

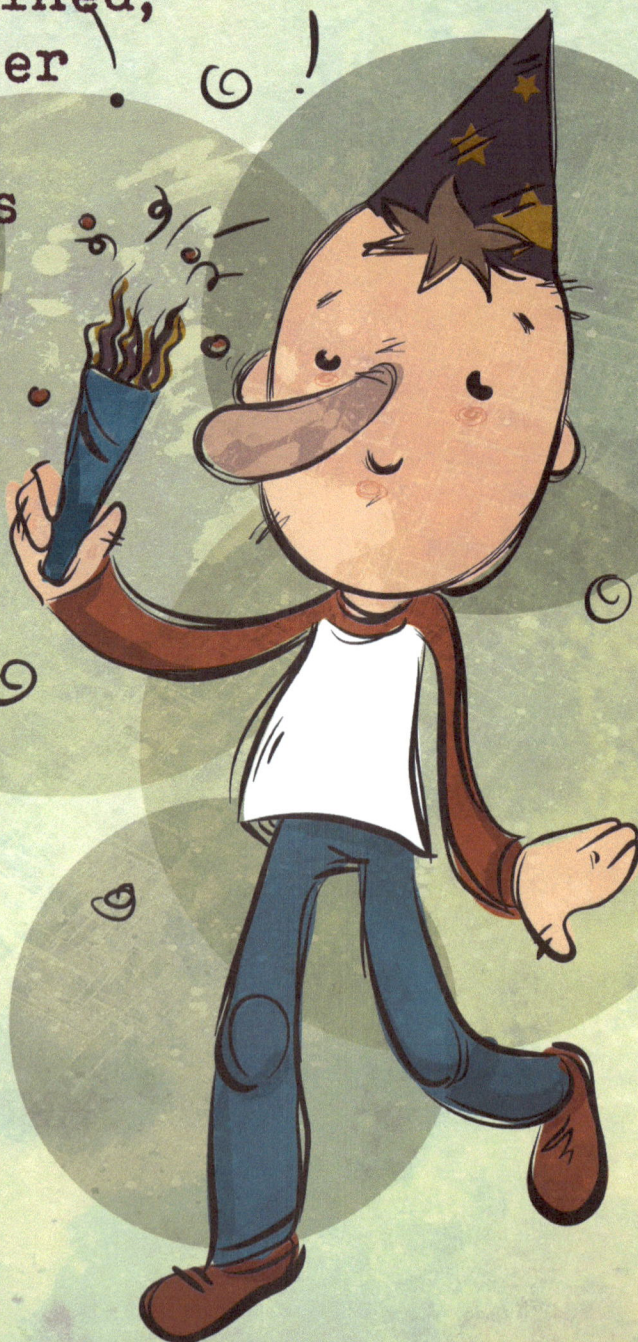

Luke and his mom brought fresh berries from the farmers market for Grandpa Charles. His mom sat next to Grandpa Charles and rubbed his upper back while he tasted the juicy berries. She wiped some of the juice that ran down his chin with a tissue. They both smiled and enjoyed the moment.

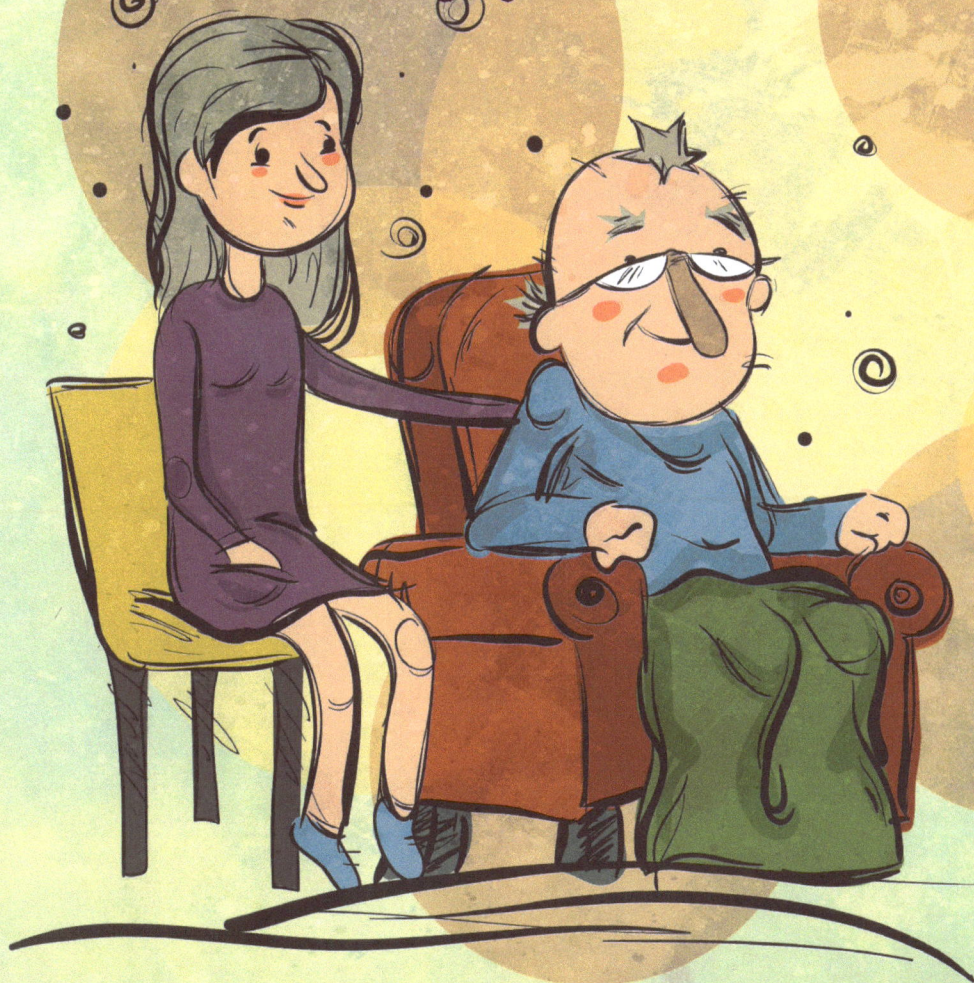

Luke was upset Grandpa Charles couldn't attend his games anymore. Suddenly he said, "I know, I can show Grandpa my new soccer skills in the courtyard at Memory Lane. I'll reenact my best plays." Luke's mother smiled and said, "That's a wonderful idea, sweetie. Your grandpa will love that."

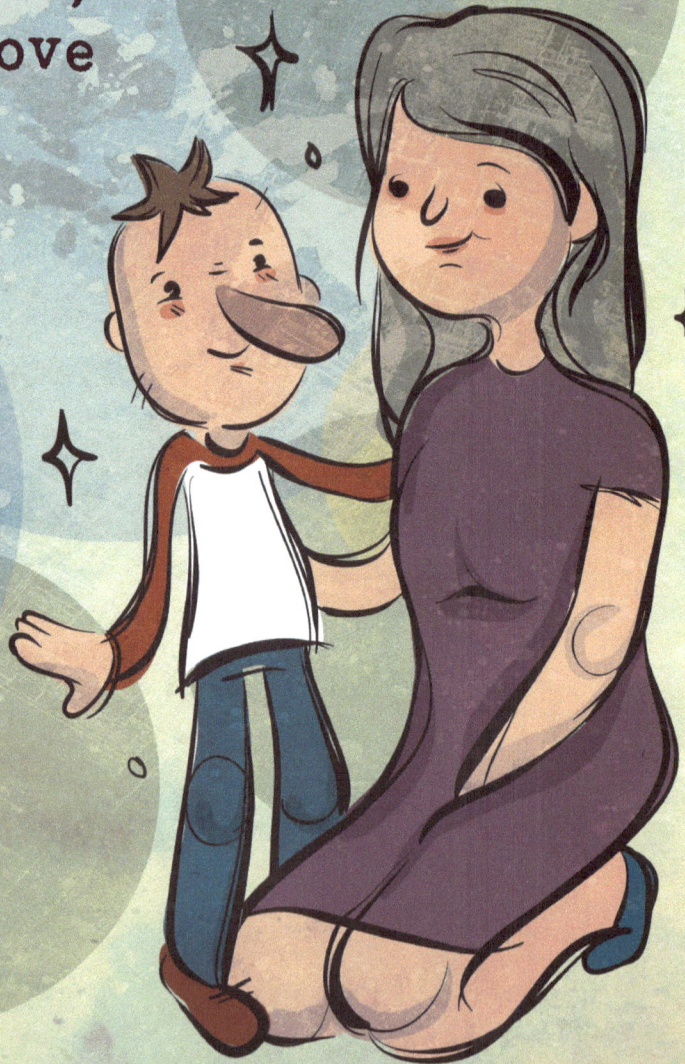

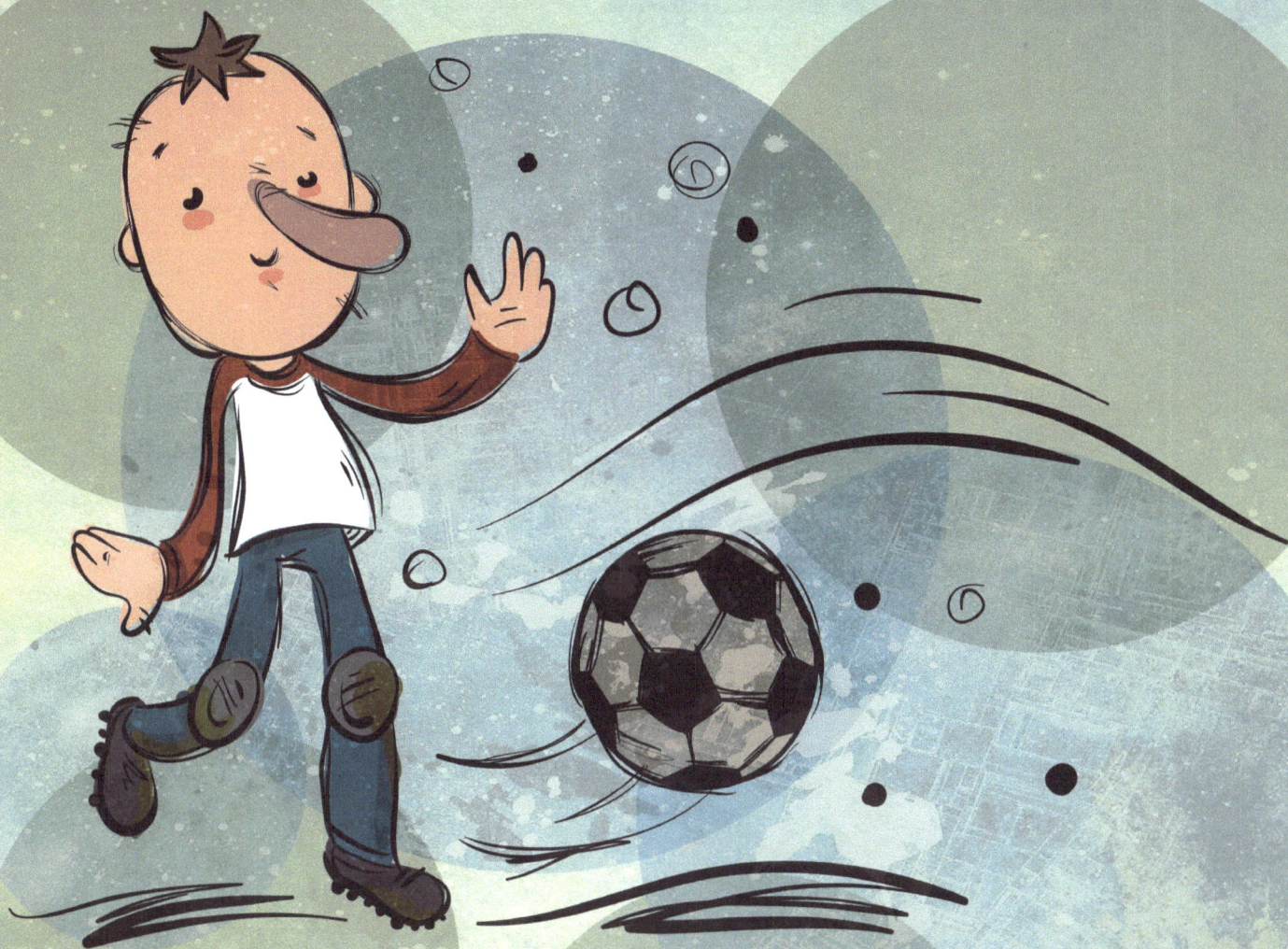

Luke provided the play by play, "First I went left, then I went right, the next thing you know, goal!" Luke turned to his grandpa and saw that he had fallen asleep. Luke joined his mother and everyone enjoyed the lovely weather.

Later that day Luke and his parents took Lilly for a walk in the park. Luke pulled four quarters from his pocket and gave one to his mom and dad. Luke tossed two quarters in the fountain. One wish was for him and one wish was for Grandpa Charles. Everyone took a moment to enjoy the tradition. It was another beautiful day at the park.

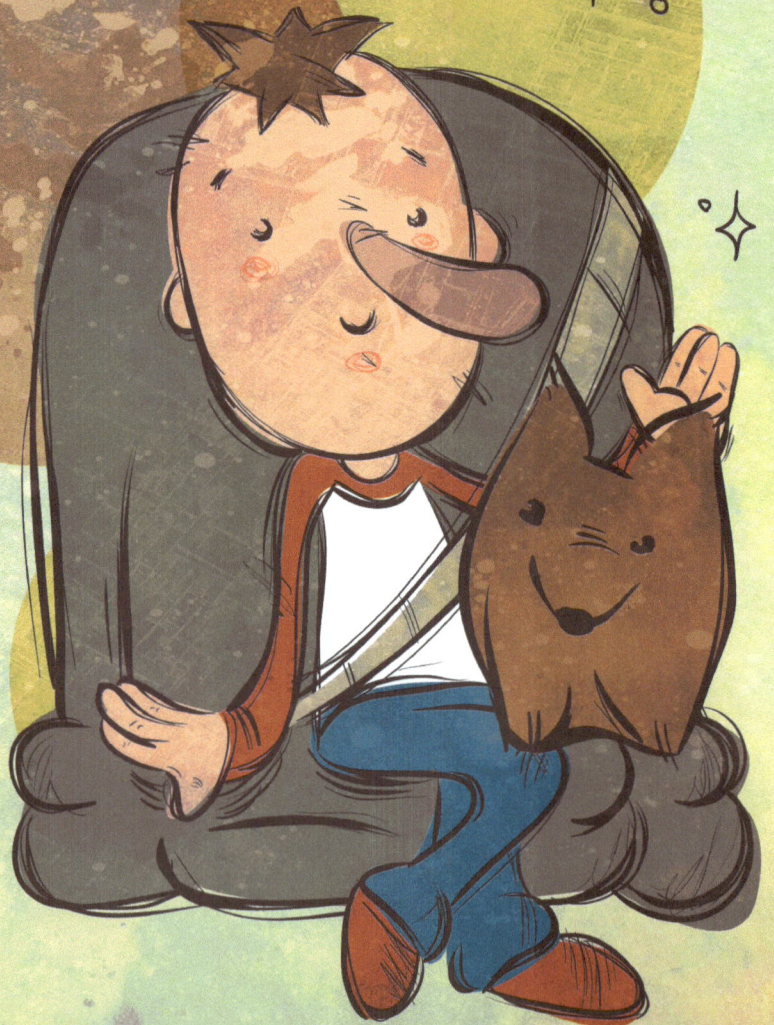

Edited by Janna Madsen

www.ingramcontent.com/pod-product-compliance
Lightning Source LLC
Chambersburg PA
CBHW060857270326
41934CB00003B/181